I EAT WHEN I'M SAD
FOOD AND FEELINGS

KIDS & OBESITY

I EAT WHEN I'M SAD
FOOD AND FEELINGS

BY RAE SIMONS

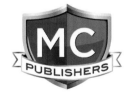

Mason Crest Publishers

MASON CREST PUBLISHERS INC.
370 Reed Road
Broomall, Pennsylvania 19008
(866)MCP-BOOK (toll free)
www.masoncrest.com

First Printing
9 8 7 6 5 4 3 2 1

Library of Congress Cataloging-in-Publication Data

Simons, Rae, 1957–
 I eat when I'm sad : food and feelings / by Rae Simons.
    p. cm. — (Obesity & kids)
 Includes bibliographical references and index.
 ISBN 978-1-4222-1714-6 (hardcover)   ISBN 978-1-4222-1705-4 (series)
 ISBN 978-1-4222-1902-7 (pbk.)   ISBN 978-1-4222-1893-8 (pbk. series)
 1. Compulsive eating—Juvenile literature. 2. Weight loss—Psychological aspects—Juvenile literature. 3. Obesity—Psychological aspects—Juvenile literature. 4. Eating disorders—Juvenile literature. I. Title.
 RC552.C65S474 2010
 616.85'26—dc22
                        2010007065

Design by MK Bassett-Harvey and Wendy Arakawa.
Produced by Harding House Publishing Service, Inc.
www.hardinghousepages.com
Cover design by Torque Advertising and Design.
Printed in USA by Bang Printing.

The creators of this book have made every effort to provide accurate information, but it should not be used as a substitute for the help and services of trained professionals.

CONTENTS

INTRODUCTION
FOR THE TEACHERS

We as a society often reserve our harshest criticism for those conditions we understand the least. Such is the case for obesity. Obesity is a chronic and often-fatal disease that accounts for 400,000 deaths each year. It is second only to smoking as a cause of premature death in the United States. People suffering from obesity need understanding, support, and medical assistance. Yet what they often receive is scorn.

Today, children are the fastest growing segment of the obese population in the United States. This constitutes a public health crisis of enormous proportions. Living with childhood obesity affects self-esteem, which down the road can affect employment and attainment of higher education. But childhood obesity is much more than a social stigma. It has serious health consequences.

Childhood obesity increases the risk for poor health in adulthood—but also even during childhood. Depression, diabetes, asthma, gallstones, orthopedic diseases, and other obesity-related conditions are all on the rise in children. Recent estimates suggest that 30 to 50 percent of children born in

2000 will develop type 2 diabetes mellitus, a leading cause of preventable blindness, kidney failure, heart disease, stroke, and amputations. Obesity is undoubtedly the most pressing nutritional disorder among young people today.

If we are to reverse obesity's current trend, there must be family, community, and national objectives promoting healthy eating and exercise. As a nation, we must demand broad-based public-health initiatives to limit TV watching, curtail junk food advertising toward children, and promote physical activity. More than rhetoric, these need to be our rallying cry. Any-thing short of this will eventually fail, and within our lifetime obesity will become the leading cause of death in the United States if not in the world. This series is an excellent first step in battling the obesity crisis by educating young children about the risks, the realities, and what they can do to build healthy lifestyles right now.

CHAPTER 1
FEEDING OUR FEELINGS

"You need to lose weight, Honey."

Amy scowled at her mom, and her face turned red. Amy's whole life, she had been hearing words like "chunky" and "solid" from her grandma, words Amy knew really meant "fat." The kids at school teased her because she wasn't good at gym

Being overweight can make it hard to keep up with other kids during recess or gym class.

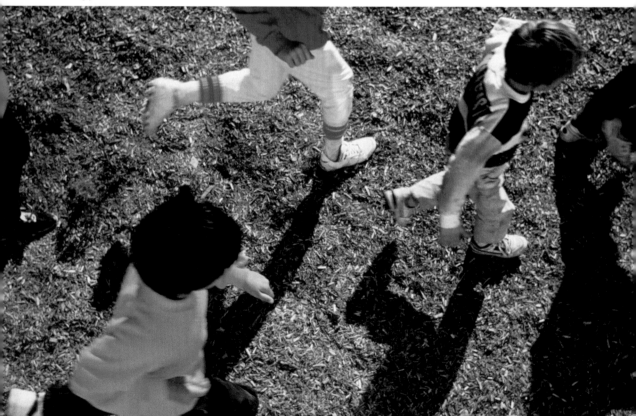

("If you weren't so big, Amy," her friend Jennifer had said to her last week, "you could run faster"), and Bobby Brown, the mean sixth-grader on the bus, called her "fatso" sometimes. But her mom had always been the one who said, "Amy, you're beautiful. You're pretty and perfect and smart, and I love you exactly the way you are." Now her mom had turned on her.

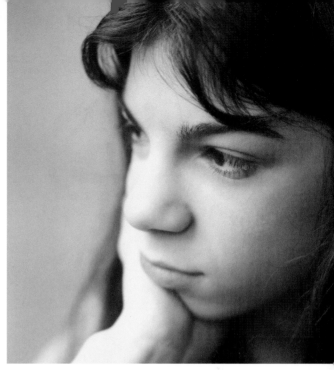

Getting teased can make you feel bad about yourself.

Amy didn't know what to say. Her eyes filled with tears and finally, she blurted, "You're mean!"

Her mom put down the book she was reading and put her arm around Amy's shoulders. "Oh Amy, I'm not being mean. I know it hurts to hear something like this. No one likes to hear they need to lose weight. But I want you to be healthy, Honey. Being overweight isn't good for you. And when you grow up, if you're heavy, it can give you serious health problems. We need to make a plan to change the way you eat. No more cookies after school—we'll have fruit and veggies instead. No more ice cream after supper, no more chips for a snack. I'll do everything I can to help you."

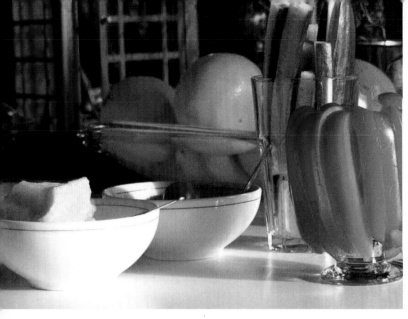

Many kids like to have a snack after school—if you do, make it a healthy choice, like fruits and veggies.

Amy stared at her mom. She felt full of upset feeling, all swirling around inside her in a cloudy mess. I don't want to go on a diet, she wanted to shout. I like food. But deep inside, she knew her mom was right.

"Okay, Amy?" Her mom gave her shoulders a squeeze. "We'll start today?"

Amy shrugged and pulled away from her mother. "Okay."

A week later, Amy trudged up the sidewalk from the bus to her house. She'd had a bad day at school. In math, they'd had a surprise quiz, and she had gotten two of the five problems wrong. Two didn't seem like so many—but the teacher had written a big red 60 on her paper, and 60 was a failing grade. Then her best friend Molly had been sick with the flu for a whole week, and Amy was left with only Jennifer and Courtney to sit with at lunch and talk to during play period. Jennifer and

Courtney liked each other better than they liked anyone else, and a lot of the time, Amy felt left out of their conversations. And worst of all, Bobby Brown had stuck out his foot on the bus as she walked down the aisle to get off at her stop. She'd tripped and fallen against the girl across the aisle. "Watch it, Hippo!" Bobby had laughed, and Amy had felt her face turn hot.

In the old days, before the diet, when Amy got inside the house, her mother would get up from her work at her desk, and then the two of them would eat cookies together and drink hot chocolate. Now, when she came through the door, she saw a tray of carrots, raw broccoli, and celery sticks waiting on the table beside a glass of water. Her mother was working at her

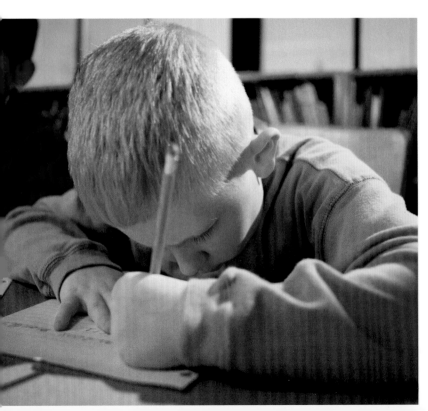

School can be hard for everyone sometimes. Ask for help when you need it and don't feel bad about yourself.

desk, writing her articles for the newspaper where she worked, and she looked too busy to be interrupted.

Amy made a face at the table and kept on walking, past her mother and up the stairs to her room.

"Don't you want a snack, Amy?" her mom called after her.

"I'm not hungry!" Amy shouted over her shoulder.

She shut her door behind her and threw herself face down on the bed. After a moment, though, she got up and knelt on the floor beside her bed. She reached underneath and pulled out the stash of Halloween candy she'd been saving.

For a long time, she sorted through the candy bars. Just the sight of them made her feel better. "I'll just have one," she whispered. She picked up each different kind of candy one by one and carefully read the weight printed on each package. Then she ate the biggest candy bar.

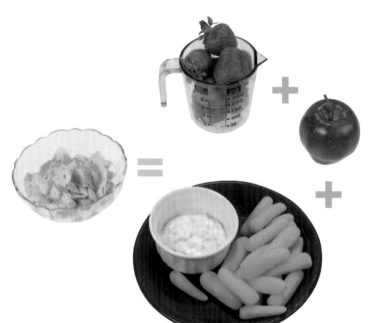

This image shows that a small bowl of chips equals the calories in a cup of strawberries, an apple and some carrot sticks with low-fat dip.

Almost at once, the sad feeling inside her began to fade away. She chewed the chocolate and caramel as slowly as she could, letting the sweetness wipe away all the day's bad moments. "Just one more," she told herself sternly as she licked chocolate off her fingertips.

By the time she had eaten two candy bars, she was ready to

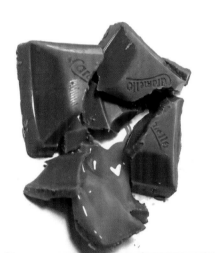

go downstairs and talk to her mom about her day. She could even smile, knowing she still had lots more candy in the plastic pumpkin under her bed. After supper, she could eat some more.

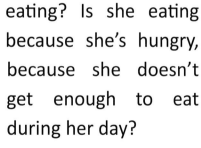

What do you think? Why is Amy eating? Is she eating because she's hungry, because she doesn't get enough to eat during her day?

No, Amy gets plenty of food. She ate breakfast before school, she ate a healthy lunch in the cafeteria with her friends, and her

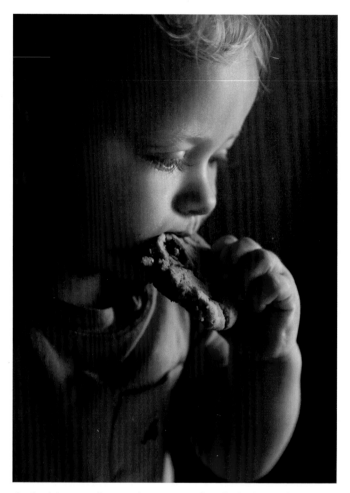

As babies we learn that some foods help us feel better when we are sad.

mother is offering her a healthy after-school snack. But Amy wants something sweet because she's had a bad day. She wants to use food to help her feel happier.

FOOD AND HAPPINESS

Amy's not the only one who depends on food to help her handle her feelings. Lots of people do, both children and grown-ups. Since the time we were very young, many of us have been taught to connect food with happiness.

Think about it. A toddler falls down and cries—and his mother gives him a cookie or a candy to stop his tears. A connection is being made in his mind between food and comfort. As he gets older, he learns that people eat to celebrate good times, like birthdays and holidays. They eat when they watch television. They eat when they get together with friends. They eat when they go to the movies. They eat at classroom parties. They eat when they go to sports events. They pretty much have special fun foods for every occasion and activity. Before long, food and good times just go together in this person's mind.

WHY DO YOU EAT?

Most of us don't always eat because we're hungry. Instead, we eat because we're bored—or frustrated —or sad—or lonely—or angry —or nervous. Our bodies need food to live, of course, but instead of feeding our bodies, we're actually feeding our feelings.

Why do you eat? Do you know?

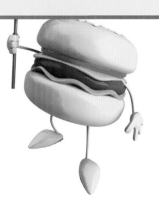

DID YOU KNOW?

One way to help you understand the reasons why you eat is to keep a food diary. Every time you want to eat something, write down how you feel. You don't even have to use words—you could just draw a happy face, a sad face, a scared face, or an angry face. Draw a circle if you're eating simply because you're hungry. When you look back at your diary after a few days, you should be able to see how often you're eating to feed your feelings.

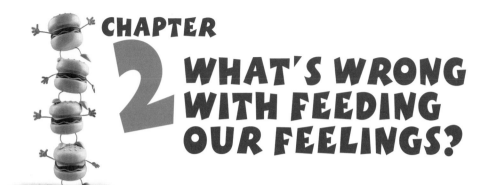

CHAPTER 2
WHAT'S WRONG WITH FEEDING OUR FEELINGS?

Food nourishes our bodies and helps keep them healthy. It tastes good. Eating is meant to be something we enjoy. People who like to cook work hard to make food that tastes good, and many people get a lot of satisfaction from preparing food. Sharing a meal with others is a time for talking and being close. All those things are good things. Food is a good thing, and eating is an important part of life.

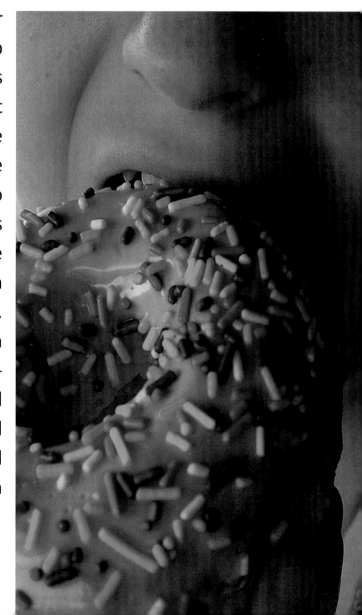

But eating because we're sad or bored or nervous isn't a good thing. When we eat because of feelings, we're not listening to our bodies' messages. Instead of eating when we're hungry and stopping when we're full, we eat when we're sad—and then we keep eating, even after our stomachs are full. Instead of eating the things our bodies need to be healthy, we tend to eat lots of sweets and starchy foods like cookies, brownies, chips, french fries, donuts, candy, crackers, and bread. These kinds of food often don't have as many **nutrients** as other foods do. When we build our eating habits around our feelings,

> **What are nutrients:** They're the things in food our bodies need to be healthy. Vitamins, carbo-hydrates, protein, fats, and minerals are all nutrients found in food.

Eating should be something you enjoy, but it is important to eat for the nutrients in food, not just for the feelings food gives you.

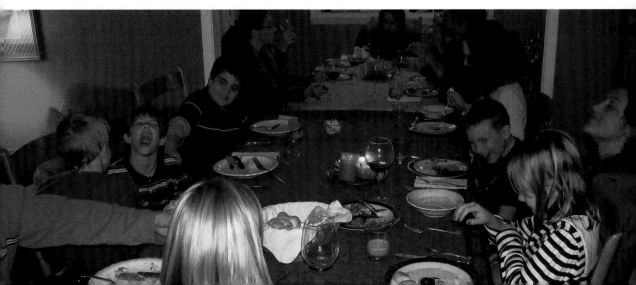

we probably aren't getting enough of the things our bodies need to be healthy. And we often end up overweight.

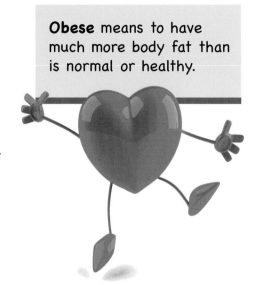

Obese means to have much more body fat than is normal or healthy.

So what's so bad about being overweight? Like Amy, lots of people in our world today are "chunky." That doesn't mean they're ugly. They may not even be truly **obese**. People come in all different sizes and shapes— and no one should ever be insulted or treated with less respect because of their weight. But as Amy's mother told her, being overweight can be dangerous. It puts you at risk for getting sick, both now, when you're still a kid, and later, when you grow up.

Children who are overweight or obese are more likely to get diabetes. This is a disease where

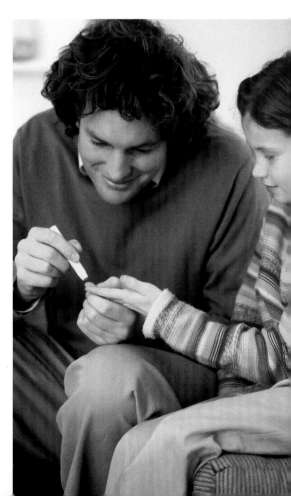

If you have diabetes, you need to test your blood sugar levels every day.

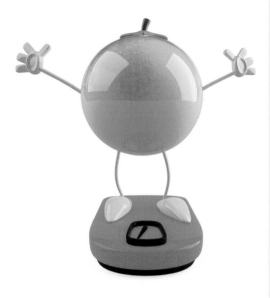

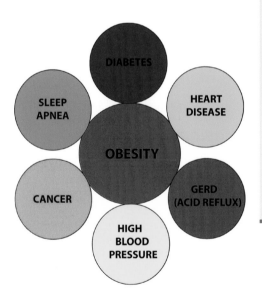

DIABETES

SLEEP APNEA

HEART DISEASE

OBESITY

CANCER

GERD (ACID REFLUX)

HIGH BLOOD PRESSURE

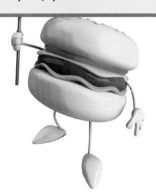

Being overweight is unhealthy in part because it can lead to so many other health problems.

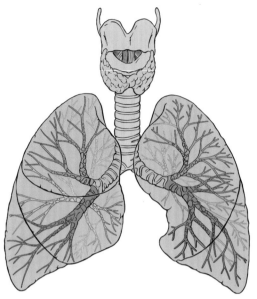

Being overweight can affect the health of your lungs since you can't run and exercise as much as you should.

DID YOU KNOW?

Even though doctors use BMI to determine if you're overweight or obese, BMI is sometimes wrong. That's because people who have lots of muscle can also weigh more, even though they don't have much fat. These two boys, for example, have the same height, same weight, and the same BMI—but one is overweight and the other one is muscular!

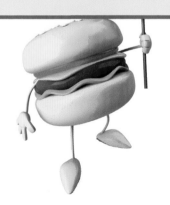

your body doesn't break down sugar the way it should. If you have diabetes, you will probably have to take medicine or have special shots every day to help your body process sugar normally. Diabetes can lead to other diseases as well, including blindness. It can make it hard for you to heal after a cut or injury.

Being overweight also increases your chances of having heart disease. This is an illness we usually connect with older people, but carrying too much weight around is hard on your heart, no matter your age. Even worse, the heavier you are, the harder it probably will be for you to run around and exercise. Your heart and lungs need exercise to be healthy. Today, more and more children are obese or overweight—and more and more children are getting heart disease.

As people who are overweight or obese grow older, the added weight on their bodies can lead to a range of diseases and problems. These can include:

- high blood pressure (which increases your chances of having a **stroke**)
- **arthritis**
- gallbladder disease
- breathing problems
- some forms of **cancers**

Being overweight can also mean that you have more problems handling your emotions. People who are obese or overweight are more likely to have **depression**. So eating

What is a stroke: A stroke is when the cells in your brain suddenly die because they don't get enough blood.

What is arthritis: Arthritis is a disease that causes your joints to be sore and stiff.

What are cancers: Cancers are a kind of disease that causes the cells in different parts of your body to grow too fast, to the point that they kill healthy cells.

What is depression: Depression is an emotional illness that makes people feel very sad most of the time.

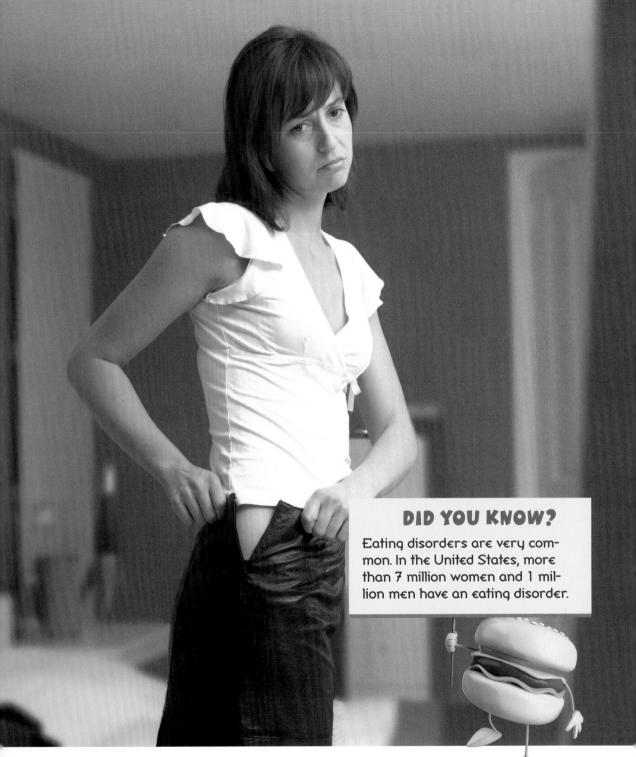

Some people eat more when they are sad about their bodies, but other people eat less and develop eating disorders.

can be a vicious circle—you eat because you feel sad, but eating too much makes you overweight, and being overweight can make you even sadder!

Sometimes people who eat to feed their feelings can go too far the other way. They feel ugly, and they start to hate their bodies for being overweight. Instead, of forming healthier eating habits, they may develop something called an eating disorder. People who have eating disorders may refuse to eat hardly anything at all, to the point that they get sick. Or they may eat and eat and eat and eat—and then make themselves throw up or go the bathroom to get rid of all the food before it can make them fat. Either kind of eating disorder can be dangerous. Eating disorders are very serious conditions that can make people very sick.

DID YOU KNOW?

Eating disorders often begin when people are children or teenagers. Of the grown-ups who have eating disorders, 10% began having this problem before they were 10 years old; 33% were between the ages of 11 and 15; 43% were between the ages of 16 and 20.

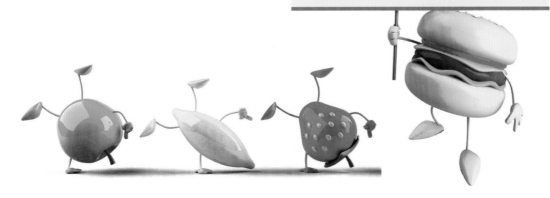

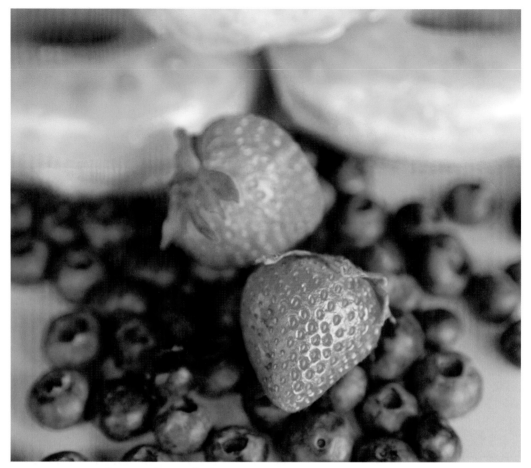

Learning to understand your feelings will help you learn to make smarter choices about your eating.

Food is good for you. But food and feelings need to be separated. That doesn't mean you should ignore your feelings, though. Your feelings are important—and so are you! That's why you need to learn to listen to what your feelings are telling you.

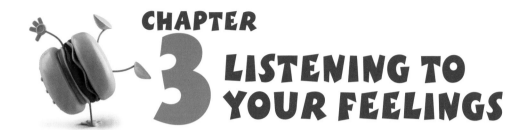

CHAPTER 3
LISTENING TO YOUR FEELINGS

"I'm a big fat pig!"

Amy shouted the words at her mother, with tears streaming down her face.

"No, you're not."

Moms want what is best for their children—even if kids sometimes feel like that is not the case.

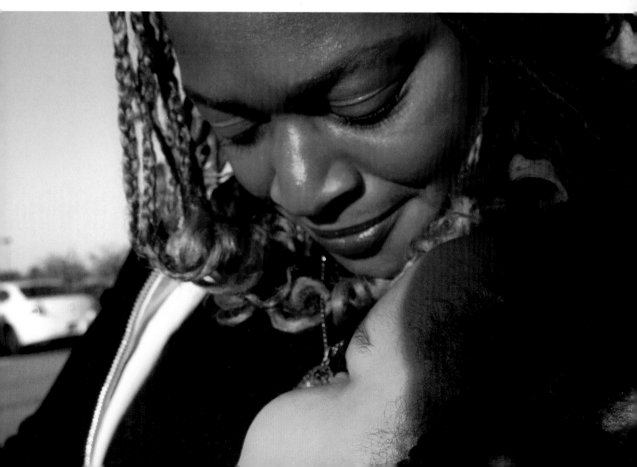

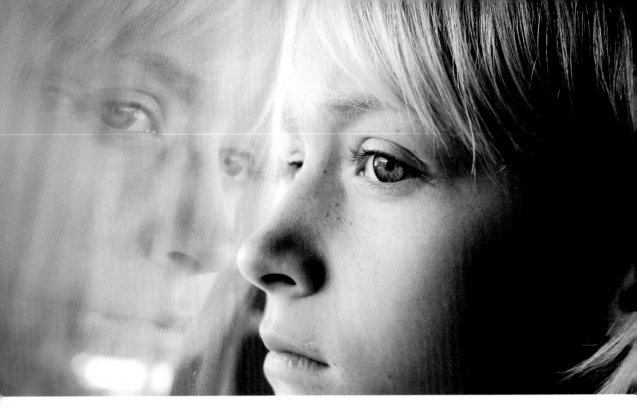

Everyone struggles with self-image sometimes.

Her mom spoke the words with such total sureness that Amy wanted to believe her. But she couldn't. "You think I'm a pig too," she spit at her mother. "If you didn't think I was, you wouldn't be making me be on a diet!"

Her mother sat down at her desk. She had a mixed-up look on her face, as though she wasn't sure what she should say or do next. In a way, Amy was happy to see her mom look like that, but in another way, it made her sad.

"Oh Amy," her mom said. "I never meant to make you think you were fat or ugly. You know how much I love you. I think you're the most beautiful, perfect ten-year-old in the whole world."

"How can you say that?" Amy sniffed. "You know I'm overweight."

"Yes, you are. But that doesn't keep you from being beautiful and smart and talented and all the other things you are. All of us have problems we have to work on. Things about ourselves we struggle with. I have them too. Everyone does." Her mom sighed and put her arm around Amy.

Amy sighed too. She let herself lean against her mom's knees, but inside, she still felt sad and upset.

Being "forced" to go on a diet can make you feel angry or upset. Find a way to express your emotions—it will make you feel better.

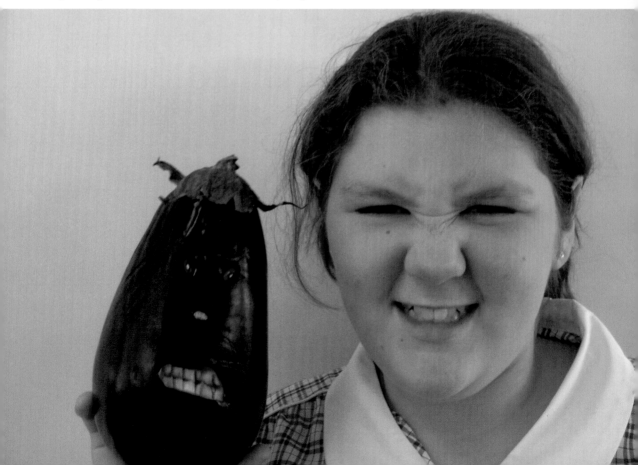

"Okay," her mom said after a moment. "Maybe we've been going about this the wrong way. It's hard for you to get used to eating differently, isn't it?"

Amy nodded.

"Well, maybe we should talk about that. How does being on a diet make you feel?"

Amy searched her mom's face, not sure what her mother wanted her to say.

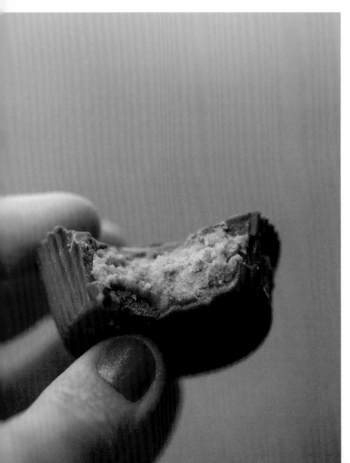

Feeling mad or sad can make you want to eat the unhealthy foods that make you feel happy.

"Just tell the truth, Amy." Her mom smiled. "I won't get mad."

"It makes ME mad," Amy blurted. "I feel like it was just something you decided for me. I didn't have any choice. I feel frustrated and mad and upset and—"

"I think I get the picture." Her mom played with a strand of Amy's hair for a moment. "I guess I don't blame you. I'd feel like that too. I'm sorry. Like I said, I went about this the wrong way. Will you forgive me?"

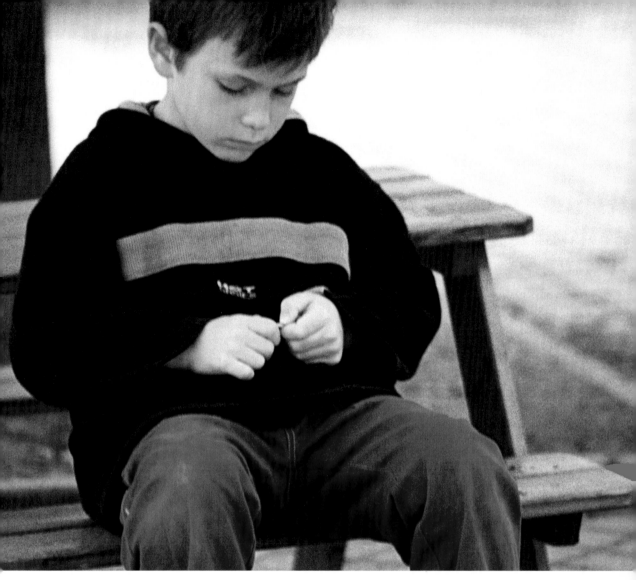

Loneliness often leads to unhealthy eating. Find someone you can talk to about it rather than eating junk food.

Amy looked up at her mother. She nodded.

"Thank you." Her mother's smile was wider this time. "So when you feel all those things—mad and frustrated and upset—what do you want to do?"

Amy bit her lip, thinking. She made a face. "It makes me want to eat. But not carrots and oranges and broccoli and salads.

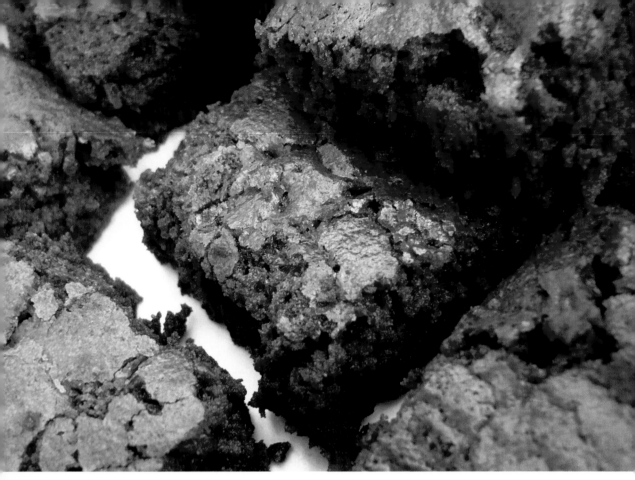

A nice fudgy brownie might make you feel better for a little while, but healthier foods, like fruits and veggies, will actually make you feel better in the long run.

It makes me want to eat candy. And chocolate chip cookies. And corn chips. And chocolate fudge brownie ice cream."

"Ah." Her mom gave a little laugh. "Well, that just makes things harder for you, doesn't it?"

Amy nodded again.

"So what can we do instead when you feel that way?"

Amy thought about her mother's words. "Could we do something together? We used to eat cookies and drink hot chocolate together after school—but now, you keep on working at your desk, and I just eat my snack alone. It makes me feel lonely."

Her mom looked sad again. "Oh, I'm sorry, Amy! That wasn't very nice of me. And what do you want to do when you feel lonely?"

Amy giggled through her tears. "I want to eat. I want to go in the kitchen and eat and eat and eat until I don't feel sad or lonely anymore."

"Well, I don't blame you! But how about if we think of something else to do together instead?" Amy's mother reached for her iPod beside her computer. She thumbed through the songs, and then loud, angry music burst out of the speakers in the living room. "Want to dance?" her mom asked.

Amy hung back for a minute. When she was little, she and her mother had loved to dance together, making up silly movements and laughing, but Amy thought maybe she was too old for that now. She watched her

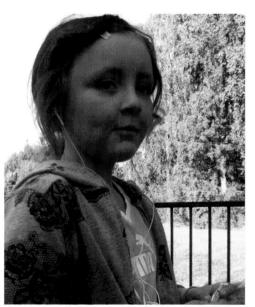

Music can be a great way to deal with your feelings—fast, happy songs might make you happier, or perhaps slow, sad songs might help you let out your sadness without turning to food.

mom jerk her head back and forth while she swiveled her hips. After a while, Amy started to giggle.

"I'm dancing all my angry feelings," her mom shouted over the music. "Come on, join me!"

Amy found herself moving to the beat of the music. She let her anger jerk through her hands and arms as they flung back and forth, and she stopped worrying if she looked silly. After all, there was no one there to see.

The angry song was followed by another angry song, and then it faded into a song so sad it made Amy want to cry. She and her mom danced the sad song with long slow sweeps of their arms, and then they danced a lonely song—and then they hugged each other and laughed. The next song was a happy one that made them jump and laugh.

When they stopped, they were both sweaty and panting. "Well, THAT was good exercise!" her mom gasped.

Exercise is an important part of being healthy, but it doesn't have to be boring. Find something that you think is fun, like Frisbee or dancing, and it won't even feel like exercise!

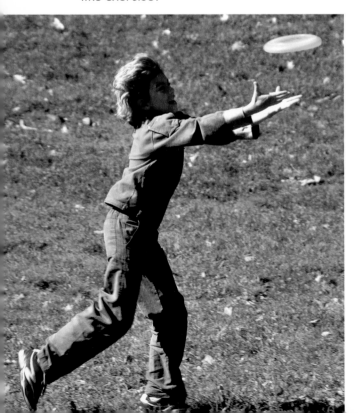

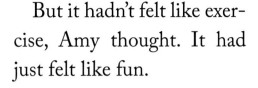

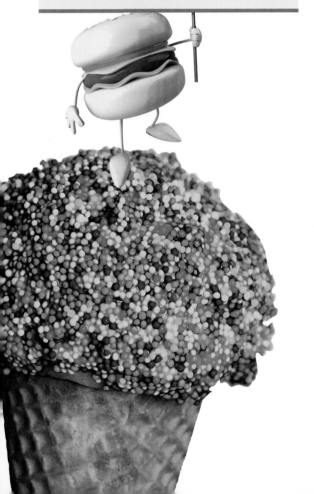

But it hadn't felt like exercise, Amy thought. It had just felt like fun.

Like Amy, most of us have feelings that are all mixed together. We may feel embarrassed and angry and lonely all at once. Sometimes, we can feel scared and excited and happy at the same time. It's often hard to sort out these feelings. Instead, of paying attention to our feelings—listening to what they're trying to tell us—we may turn to food to help us calm down.

Eating sweets makes you feel good for a reason—the sugar in food like this ice cream cone sends a "happy" message to your brain.

WHAT'S THE CONNECTION BETWEEN FOOD AND FEELINGS?

Eating is a way to do something that seems nice for yourself when you feel as though no one else is being nice enough to you. It's a way to fill up time when you're bored. And eating makes changes inside your body that can also change your emotions.

When you feel happy, your body is sending special chemicals into your brain that creates that happy feeling. Being nervous or scared makes our bodies crave more of these chemicals. So does being sad. Many things can cause these chemicals to be made, and food is one of them. So when you eat something sweet, you really do feel happier for a little while, because the sugar tells your body to send these happy chemicals into your brain. And if you didn't eat at all (if you skipped a meal or two), your emotions as well as your body would soon be upset until you gave your body food again.

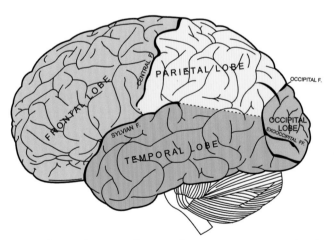

Sugar is actually very important to your brain—it helps your brain grow and helps you learn and think better. However, the best sugar comes from healthy foods, like fresh fruits.

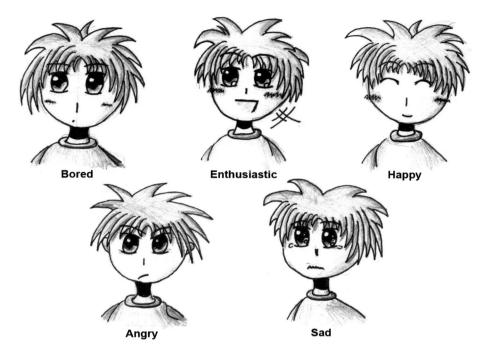

Bored   **Enthusiastic**   **Happy**

Angry   **Sad**

Learn how to identify your feelings to help learn how to stop eating when you are sad or angry.

Your body NEEDS food to be healthy, physically and emotionally. Food is a good thing. But it's not always the answer to your feelings.

That's why it's important to listen to your feelings. Instead of thinking that every feeling you have means, "I'm hungry, I need to find something to eat," pay attention to why

DID YOU KNOW?

Exercise produces the same "happy chemicals" that eating can. The more you exercise—even if it's just going for a walk—the happier you'll feel.

you want to eat. Are you really hungry? (If you are, then you need to find something healthy to fill your stomach.) Or are you bored? Sad? Lonely? Nervous?

What does identify mean? It means to give something a name, to be able to recognize something for what it really is.

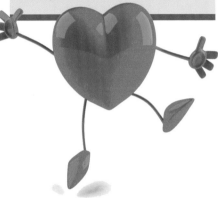

Once you can stop to **identify** what you're feeling, you've already taken the first step to break the habit of connecting food to feelings. If you're eating because you're lonely, try calling a friend on the phone or talking to a family member. Even spending time with the family pet will help. And if there's no one at all you can talk to, try writing in a journal or drawing pictures. Be your own friend. Sometimes, it's even okay to talk to yourself! If you're eating because you're sad, do something else you enjoy to help cheer yourself (listen to music, read a good book, do a hobby, play a game with someone, dance, draw a picture, go for a walk). If you're angry or frustrated, find someone you can talk to who will listen to your feelings and understand. And if there isn't anyone to listen, express your angry or frustrated feelings some other way (play a musical instrument, draw a picture, write a poem, dance, go swimming). If you're scared or nervous, think about what's scaring you. Is it something you can do something about? For

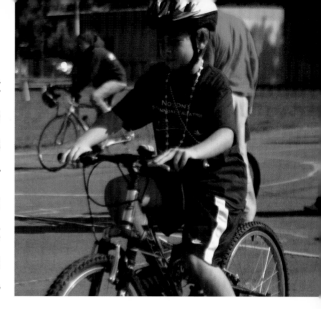

example, if you're nervous about a big test, then studying will help you feel more confident. If it's something you can't control—for instance, your mother says you have to go to the doctor to get shots—find something besides food to distract you from your fear (read an exciting book, talk to one of your favorite people, play a game that requires a lot of attention, watch something interesting on television).

A fun activity or hobby can make you feel happier, and it is much healthier than eating when you are sad or angry.

Food is a healthy and necessary part of life—but eating will never solve our problems. It may give us some **temporary** relief, but before long, our sad, nervous, angry feelings will be right back.

Feelings are important, though, so pay attention to them. Don't try to pretend you're not feeling something you really are feeling. Instead, practice really listening to your feelings.

What does temporary mean? It means that something only lasts for a while. Eventually, whatever it is will come to an end, because it's not permanent.

Hear what they're saying to you. And then do something to help, the way you would if your best friend asked you for something.

Be a good friend to yourself. Listen to your feelings.

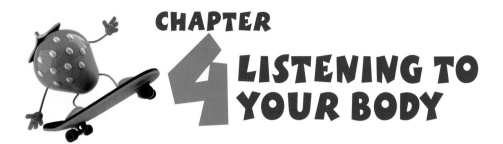

Your body needs to eat. You can't walk or run, talk or think without the **energy** you get from food.

MEASURING FOOD'S ENERGY

You've probably heard people talk about calories. Sometimes it may sound as though calories are bad things. After all, commercials are always making low-calorie foods sound as though they're healthier, and people who are trying to lose weight will count their calories. It's true that too many calories can make us fat—but we also need calories.

What is energy?
Energy is the ability to be active, the power it takes to move your body.

We use inches and feet (or centimeters and meters) to measure how long or tall something is; we use pints and quarts (or liters) to measure liquids like milk and soda—and we use calories to measure how much energy is in a certain food.

Each one of us needs a certain amount of calories every day to be healthy and have the energy we need to do all the things we do. Even sitting still takes a certain number of calories, but the more active we are, the more calories we need. People who are bigger, active, or who are growing usually need more calories than smaller people, people who don't move around very much, and people who aren't growing.

When we eat more calories than we need, our bodies store the extra energy as fat. Long ago, our ancestors went through times when they had plenty of food, followed by times when food was scarcer. Their bodies' stores of fat helped them get through the times when they had less food. Today, though, many times our bodies just keep storing more and more fat that never needs to be used. When that happens, we end up being overweight or obese.

To get rid of these extra stores of fat, we need to do one of two things: take in fewer calories, forcing our bodies to use up the stored

Recommended Daily Calories		
Age	**Boys**	**Girls**
2	1000	1000
3	1000–1400	1000–1200
4–5	1200–1400	1200–1400
6	1400–1600	1200–1400
7	1400–1600	1200–1600
8	1400–1600	1400–1600
9	1600–1800	1400–1600
10	1600–1800	1400–1800
11	1800–2000	1600–1800
12	1800–2200	1600–2000
13	2000–2200	1600–2000
14	2000–2400	1800–2000
15	2200–2600	1800–2000
16–18	2400–2800	1800–2000
19–20	2600–2800	2000–2200

Everybody has different calorie needs.

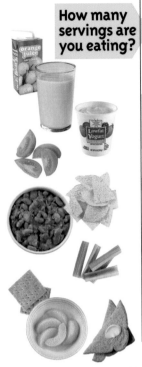

How many servings are you eating?

Nutrition Facts
Serving Size 1 cup (228g)
Servings Per Container 2

Amount Per Serving

Calories 250   Calories from Fat 110

	% Daily Value*
Total Fat 12g	18%
Saturated Fat 3g	15%
Trans fat 0g	
Cholesterol 30mg	10%
Sodium 470mg	20%
Total Carbohydrate 31g	10%
Dietary Fiber 0g	0%
Sugars 5g	
Protein 5g	

Vitamin A	4%	•	Vitamin C	2%
Calcium	20%	•	Iron	4%

* Percent Daily Values are based on a 2,000 calorie diet. Your daily values may be higher or lower depending on your calorie needs:

	Calories:	2,000	2,500
Total Fat	Less than	65g	80g
Sat Fat	Less than	20g	25g
Cholesterol	Less than	300mg	300mg
Sodium	Less than	2,400mg	2,400mg
Total Carbohydrate		300g	375g
Dietary Fiber		25g	30g

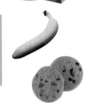

Get What You Need!

Get LESS

5 % or less is low

20 % or more is high

Get ENOUGH

5 % or less is low

20 % or more is high

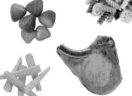

What's the Best Choice for You?
Use the Nutrition Facts Label to Make Choices

Nutrition labels give a lot of information that can help you choose the healthiest foods.

energy in our fat—or use up more calories by exercising more, which will also make our bodies use up the fat we've stored. The best way to lose weight, experts tell us, is to do both: cut back on calories and exercise more.

DID YOU KNOW?

An athlete like a bicyclist who is in training for a big race may need to eat as many as 6,000 calories a day.

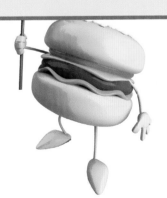

All foods have calories, whether it's cookies or carrots, lettuce or ice cream, but some foods have more calories than others. This means that if you ate a pound of lettuce, you would have eaten only about 80 calories (and you would have had to eat about 16 cups of lettuce)—but if you ate a pound of chocolate chip cookies (about 10 cookies), you would have eaten 2,100 calories! That's a big difference.

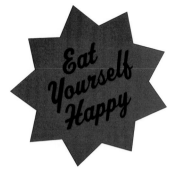

Eat Yourself Happy

The foods that have lots of calories (like cookies and candy) also often have fewer nutrients (the things in food your body needs to be healthy)—and yet these are often the foods we most crave when we're trying to feed our feelings instead of our bodies. Sugary foods (like desserts and candy) and starchy foods (like bread, french fries, macaroni, and pancakes) fill our bodies with a rush of the "happy chemicals" we talked about in the last chapter—but the rush doesn't last.

DID YOU KNOW?

Scientists have discovered the best combination of foods your body needs to be healthy. A diagram of this combination looks like a pyramid, with the foods you need to eat more at the bottom, and the foods you need to eat less at the top. The U.S. Department of Agriculture, the part of the American government that deals with food, farming, and nutrition, has created a picture called "MyPyramid" to help you understand better how much and what kinds of foods you need to eat in order to be healthy.

Before long, our feelings crash, and we're once again craving more of those sugary or starchy foods to give ourselves another rush of good feelings.

THE BEST WAY TO BE HEALTHY

Experts say that dieting really isn't the best approach to losing weight. People may lose weight on a diet, but after a while, most people feel like Amy did—frustrated and resentful—and they go back to eating the way they did before. Sometimes they eat even more than they did before.

The best way to lose weight and be healthy is to change the way you think about food. Feed your body when it's hungry. Give it the foods it needs to be healthy. Find fun ways to get more exercise, which will also help keep your body healthier. Get plenty of sleep.

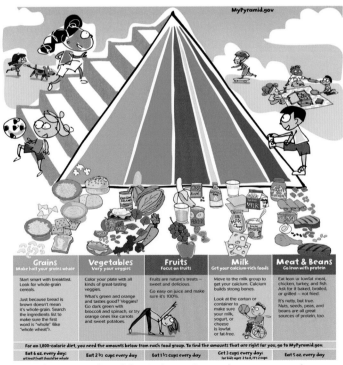

Part of getting healthy is learning why you eat, but you also need to learn what to eat and how much to eat.

Be patient with yourself. It takes time to change the way we think. Losing weight isn't easy. Amy will need her mom's help—and her mom will need to learn the best way to help her. Her mother wants Amy to lose weight because she loves Amy—but do you think her mom has made any mistakes so far? Do you think that together, Amy and her mom will find new ways to think about food and exercise?

Amy will probably get discouraged sometimes and fall back into old habits. Kids may say unkind things to her that hurt her feelings. We all have things like that happen to us, and it's easy to get upset with ourselves, to start not liking ourselves because we don't act or look the way we wished.

But losing weight because you don't like yourself never works very well. When we don't like ourselves, we feel sad and angry—and those feelings just make us want to eat more. Instead, try making a list of all the things that make you special. And then think about losing weight as something you do for yourself, so that you have more energy to do all those special things. Learn to eat because you are listening to your body. And at the same time, learn to listen to your feelings too. Give your feelings what they really need, instead of food. Change the way you live—because you're worth it.

Be your own best friend!

READ MORE ABOUT IT

Abramovitz, Melissa. *Diseases & Disorders: Obesity.* Farmington Hills, Mich.: Lucent, 2004.

Chilman-Blair, Kim. *What's Up with Pam?* New York: Rosen, 2010.

Gay, Kathlyn. *Am I Fat?* Berkeley Heights, N.J.: Enslow, 2006.

Jimerson, M. N. *Childhood Obesity.* Farmington Hills, Mich.: Lucent, 2008.

Johnson, Susan and Laurel Mellin. *Just for Kids! Obesity Prevention*. San Anselmo, Calif.: Balboa, 2002.

Olson, Judith K. *I Can Hardly Wait.* Parker, Colo.: Outskirts, 2006.

Prim-Ed. *Lifestyle Choices*. Boston: Prim-Ed, 2005.

Watson, Stephanie. *The Genetics of Obesity.* New York: Rosen, 2008.

FIND OUT MORE ON THE INTERNET

Comfort Eating
www.blubberbuster.com/board/
emotional_eating.htm

Emotional Eating
kidshealth.org/teen/food_fitness/
dieting/emotional_eating.html

Empowered Kids
www.treatingeatingdisorders.com/
empoweredkidz/

Family Food Experts
betterfoodchoices.info

The Food Guide Pyramid
kidshealth.org/kid/stay_healthy/food/
pyramid.html

Healthy Food Choices: Nutrition Explorations
www.nutritionexplorations.org/parents/
health-food.asp

MyPyramid for Kids
www.mypyramid.gov/Kids/

INDEX

PICTURE CREDITS

ABOUT THE AUTHOR

Rae Simons has ghostwritten several adult books on dieting and obesity. She is also the author of more than thirty young adult books. She lives in upstate New York, where she tries hard to get enough exercise and eat healthy foods.